82 Alzheimer's Preventing Meal and Juice Recipes:

Reduce the Risk of Alzheimer's Disease by Using Vitamin and Mineral Specific Foods!

By

Joe Correa CSN

COPYRIGHT

This publication is designed to provide accurate and authoritative information regarding the subject matter covered. It is sold with the understanding that neither the author nor the publisher is engaged in rendering medical advice. If medical advice or assistance is needed, consult with a doctor. This book is considered a guide and should not be used in any way detrimental to your health. Consult with a physician before starting this nutritional plan to make sure it's right for you.

ACKNOWLEDGEMENTS

This book is dedicated to my friends and family that have had mild or serious illnesses so that you may find a solution and make the necessary changes in your life.

82 Alzheimer's Preventing Meal and Juice Recipes:

Reduce the Risk of Alzheimer's Disease by Using Vitamin and Mineral Specific Foods!

By

Joe Correa CSN

CONTENTS

Copyright

Acknowledgements

About The Author

Introduction

82 Alzheimer's Preventing Meal and Juice Recipes: Reduce the Risk of Alzheimer's Disease by Using Vitamin and Mineral Specific Foods!

Additional Titles from This Author

ABOUT THE AUTHOR

After years of research, I honestly believe in the positive effects that proper nutrition can have over the body and mind. My knowledge and experience has helped me live healthier throughout the years and which I have shared with family and friends. The more you know about eating and drinking healthier, the sooner you will want to change your life and eating habits.

Nutrition is a key part in the process of being healthy and living longer so get started today. The first step is the most important and the most significant.

INTRODUCTION

82 Alzheimer's Preventing Meal and Juice Recipes: Reduce the Risk of Alzheimer's Disease by Using Vitamin and Mineral Specific Foods!

By Joe Correa CSN

Alzheimer's disease, unfortunately, doesn't have a cure. However, there are some treatments for the symptoms that will not stop but will slow down the disease from progressing and improve the quality of life.

Processed foods with lots of sugar, lack of vitamins and minerals, and trans fats are some of the habits that have the ability to harm your body in ways you can't even imagine. These poor diet habits directly weaken the entire body reducing brain functions.

In order to prevent and reduce the risks of Alzheimer's disease, it's crucial to change your lifestyle and improve your diet. Brain-friendly foods like green leafy vegetables, nuts, berries, beans, whole grains, fish, and olive oil should be on your daily menu.

The diet change is simple. Increasing consumption of omega-3s, vitamins A, B, C, E, and K, and foods rich in folate, phosphorous, magnesium, and selenium. These foods include nuts, seeds, leafy greens, and fish.

The meal and juice recipes in this book will improve your health and your Alzheimer's condition in a short period of time. Try them all and see which ones are your favorite recipes.

82 ALZHEIMER'S PREVENTING MEAL AND JUICE RECIPES: REDUCE THE RISK OF ALZHEIMER'S DISEASE BY USING VITAMIN AND MINERAL SPECIFIC FOODS!

MEALS

1. Chicken, Olives, and Tomato with Spinach Herb Orzo

Combining olives, tomatoes, and spinach in this entrée create a powerhouse of anti-inflammatory agents. Increasing blood flow and providing brain cells with the oxygen they need, each of these ingredients should be consumed on a regular basis.

Ingredients:

- 1 tablespoon olive oil
- 1 tablespoon lemon juice
- 1 tablespoon dried oregano
- 1 clove garlic, minced
- 2 boneless skinless chicken breast

- 1 tomato, diced

- 1/4 cup black olives

- 2 cups orzo, cooked

- 1/2 cup spinach

- 1 teaspoon fresh basil, chopped

- 1 teaspoon fresh rosemary, chopped

How to prepare:

Combine oil, lemon juice, oregano and garlic. Pour over chicken. Chill for 30 minutes

In skillet on medium heat, place chicken. Cook the first side just until brown, flip. While cooking second side add tomatoes and olives. Gently stir without flipping chicken. Once chicken is cook through, remove from heat.

In second pan, add orzo, spinach, basil, and rosemary. Cook until spinach is wilted and orzo heated through. Spoon on to serving plate. Top with chicken, tomato, and olives.

Nutritional information:

Total calories: 675

Vitamins: Vitamin B6 1.4mg, Vitamin K 70µg

Minerals: Phosphorus 569mg, Selenium 97mg, Zinc 3mg, Thiamin 0.6mg, Riboflavin 0.5mg, Niacin 30mg, Choline 189mg

Sugars: 3g

2.   One Pot Taco Skillet

Combining black beans and brown rice produce a complete protein. A complete protein contains all nine amino acids, which prevents brain shrinkage. This simple recipe will keep you full while ensuring a multitude of nutrition and will keep your brain healthy and strong!

Ingredients:

- 1/2 pound extra lean ground beef
- 1/2 cup cooked black beans
- 1 cup salsa, preferably homemade
- 2 cups long grain brown rice, cooked
- 1/4 cup shredded cheddar cheese
- 1 tablespoon fresh cilantro, chopped

How to prepare:

In a large nonstick skillet, cook ground beef until cooked through, breaking up the meat as you go. Drain off any access fat. Add beans and salsa, allow to simmer until beans are hot. Add cooked rice. Simmer until mix thickens slightly as the moisture from the salsa cooks off.

Remove from the heat and toss in cheddar cheese. Top with chopped cilantro, if desired.

Nutritional information:

Total calories: 263

Vitamins: Vitamin A 25µg, B-6 0.4mg, B-12 1.4µg,

Minerals: Copper 218 µg, Iron 2mg, Magnesium 71mg, Niacin 5mg, Phosphorus 245mg, Selenium 20µg, Zinc 4mg

Sugars 2g

3.   Vegetable Packed Lasagna Rolls

A variety of vegetables make this lasagna entree full of vitamins and minerals to keep your brain alert and active. Each roll is the perfect serving size for an individual dinner or an addition to a family meal.

Ingredients:

- 1 (24 ounce) marinara sauce, preferably homemade
- 1 tablespoon olive oil
- 1 medium yellow onion, sliced
- 1 1/2 cups broccoli, chopped
- 1 cup mushrooms, minced
- Kosher or sea salt to taste
- 2 cloves garlic, minced
- 1 cups kale, chopped
- 1 1/2 cup ricotta cheese
- 1 1/2 cups shredded mozzarella
- 1 egg white
- 1 teaspoon fresh oregano, chopped
- 1 teaspoon fresh basil, chopped
- 1/2 teaspoon black pepper

- 12 whole wheat lasagna noodles, cooked

- 1/4 cup grated parmesan cheese

How to prepare:

Preheat oven to 425 degrees. Coat a 13" x 9" x 2" casserole dish with non-stick spray and spread 1 1/4 cups of marinara on the bottom of the dish.

In a large skillet, add oil and heat on medium-low. Sauté onion until onions are soft and begin to brown. Add broccoli, mushrooms, and pinch of salt. Mushrooms will begin to release water, cook until this water evaporates, about 2 to 3 minutes. Add garlic and kale, sauté until kale is wilted, about 3 minutes. Remove from heat and cool.

In a large mixing bowl, combine ricotta, 1 cup mozzarella, cottage cheese, egg white, oregano, basil, and pepper.

On a work surface lined with parchment paper, arrange lasagna noodles flat, add 1/4 cup cheese mix, spread evenly to cover noodles. On top of the cheese, evenly spread 1/4 cup of cooked vegetables. Start rolling the noodle at the end closest to you. Place lasagna rolls seam side down, not quite touching, in the prepared casserole dish. Evenly spread 1 cup marinara over rolls, sprinkle with remaining mozzarella and parmesan.

Cover with aluminum foil and bake 20 minutes, or until cheese is hot and bubbly. If desired, serve rolls with additional heated marinara.

Nutritional information:

Total calories: 532

Vitamins: Vitamin A 413µg, B-6 0.6mg, B-12 1.4µg, Vitamin C 76mg, Vitamin K 300µg

Minerals: Copper 850 µg, Iron 4mg, Magnesium 97mg, Niacin 9mg, Phosphorus 599mg, Selenium 46µg, Zinc 4mg

Sugars 12g

4. One Pan Chicken and Broccoli

Loaded with vitamins C and K, this easy one pan dinner helps increase energy, reduce your risk of stroke, and improve memory! Broccoli makes this a powerful anti-oxidant rich entrée anyone can enjoy.

Ingredients:

- 4 cups broccoli florets
- 4 tablespoons water
- 2 boneless and skinless free-range chicken breast
- 1 clove garlic, smashed and minced
- 1/2 teaspoon dry thyme
- 1/4 teaspoon ground rosemary
- 1/2 teaspoon ground sage
- Kosher salt
- Ground black pepper

How to prepare:

Preheat oven to 375 degrees.

Lightly spray baking sheet with non-stick spray. Place the broccoli evenly on the baking sheet and drizzle water on top   of   broccoli.

On top of the broccoli, place chicken breast. Sprinkle remaining ingredients on top of chicken.

Bake 15 to 20 minutes until chicken reaches an internal temperature of 165 degrees and no pink remains.

Nutritional information:

Total calories: 178

Vitamins: B-6 1mg, Vitamin C 96mg, Vitamin K 118µg

Minerals: Potassium 664mg, Niacin 9mg, Phosphorus 271mg, Selenium 31µg

Sugars 0g

5.   Capresse Stuffed Portabella Mushroom

High in vitamin E, this stuffed portabella mushroom is the ultimate brain protector. The most potent of all amino acids, vitamin E allows body and brain to return to normality and protects the body and brain from stress while providing energy.

Ingredients:

- 3 tablespoons extra virgin olive oil, divided
- 1 garlic clove, minced
- 2 large portabella mushrooms, stems and insides removed
- Kosher salt
- 1/2 cup spinach
- 1 cup tomatoes, diced
- 2 ounces' fresh part skim mozzarella cheese
- 2 teaspoons balsamic vinegar
- 1 tablespoon fresh basil, chopped

How to prepare:

Preheat oven to 350 degrees.

Combine two tablespoons of olive oil and garlic. Brush on

inside and outside of portabella mushrooms, sprinkle with salt.

In sauté pan, heat remaining olive oil on medium heat. Sauté spinach until wilted. Spoon half the spinach into each mushroom. Top with diced tomato followed by mozzarella.

Place filled mushrooms on cooking sheet sprayed with non-stick cooking spray. Bake for 15 to 20 minutes until cheese is melted and beginning to bubble. Mushrooms should be soft. Drizzle with balsamic vinegar and sprinkle with chopped basil

Nutritional information:

Total calories: 310

Vitamins: Vitamin D 9µg, Vitamin E 4mg, Vitamin K 62µg

Minerals: Phosphorus 223mg, Selenium 21µg, Niacin 5mg

Sugars 6g

6.   Turkey Burger with Avocado Relish

Avocados contain the right combination of healthy fats and vitamins to encourage and improve cognitive brain function; including memory and concentration. Supporting healthy blood flow, avocados also help improve cholesterol and can prevent strokes. Topping this juicy turkey burger with fresh avocado relish is not only creamy and delicious, but healthy brain food!

Ingredients:

- 6 ounces ground turkey
- Pinch of cayenne pepper (more if spicier is desired)
- 1/4 teaspoon smoky paprika
- Kosher salt
- 1/2 avocado
- 2 tablespoons onion, minced
- 1 tablespoon jalapeno, minced
- 2 teaspoons fresh lime juice
- 1 tablespoon fresh cilantro, chopped
- 1 whole wheat hamburger bun
- 1 slice Monterey jack cheese
- 1/4 cup fresh baby arugula

How to prepare:

Light and heat grill to medium low heat.

In small bowl, lightly mix turkey, cayenne, paprika, and salt. Form into a patty no more than 3/4 inches thick. Press thumb in center of patty so the burger will not bulge in the middle. Lightly spray each side of the burger with non-stick spray. Place on grill and grill each side approximately 6 minutes or until no pink remains in the center.

For the avocado relish, lightly mash avocado. The avocado should be creamy but slightly lumpy. Add onion, jalapeno, lime juice, and cilantro. Mix until combined.

To assemble, place burger on bun. Top with cheese, avocado relish, and arugula. Serve.

Nutritional information:

Total calories: 304

Vitamins: Vitamin B6 .4mg, Vitamin B12 1µg

Minerals: Phosphorus 280mg, Selenium 32µg, Niacin 6mg, Zinc 3mg, Riboflavin 0.3mg

Sugars 3g

7. Green beans with shitake mushroom in lemon garlic sauce

Green beans contain high amount of fiber which is beneficial in improving intestinal health, preventing heart disease and certain cancers. Regulated blood sugar and lower cholesterol levels will benefit your brain immensely.

Ingredients:

- 3 cups Green beans, cut into 1"
- 2 Tbsp. Garlic
- ½ cup Shallots, thinly sliced
- ½ cup Shitake mushrooms, sliced thinly
- ¼ cup Olive oil
- 2 Tbsp. Lemon juice
- 1/8 tsp. Salt
- 1/8 tsp. Pepper

How to prepare:

Over medium heat, heat the olive oil and stir in the garlic, shallots, shitake mushrooms and green beans. Stir-fry for 3 minutes or until garlic and shallots are brown and tender. Add the lemon juice and season with salt and pepper. Remove from heat, transfer to a plate and enjoy!

Serving Size 292 g

Nutritional information:

Total calories 332

Vitamin A 32%, Vitamin C 66%, Calcium 9%, Iron 14%

Sugars 4.0g

8.   One Pack Shrimp Bake

While the spices add a depth of flavor to this easy One Pack Shrimp Bake, the shrimp and spinach add essential Omega 3's and Vitamins. These Omega 3's and Vitamins provide increased blood flow, providing the brain with oxygen; promoting memory and concentration. Astaxanthin found in shrimp reduces the risk of brain inflammatory disease.

Ingredients:

- 1/2 teaspoon garlic powder
- 1/2 teaspoon smoked Paprika
- 1/4 teaspoon cayenne pepper
- 1/2 teaspoon dried oregano
- 1/4 teaspoon ground thyme
- 1/4 teaspoon Kosher salt
- 2 pounds' raw large wild caught shrimp, peeled and deveined
- 2 cups baby spinach leaves
- 1 medium yellow onion, cut into quarters
- 2 large tomatoes, cut into quarters
- 1 pound baby red potatoes, halved
- 2 tablespoons olive oil

- 1/2 cup water

- 2 tablespoons chopped fresh parsley leaves

How to prepare:

Preheat oven to 425 degrees

Combine garlic, paprika, cayenne pepper, oregano, thyme, and salt. Mix well and set aside.

Cut turkey sausage into pieces, each about 1 inch long.

Cut four sheets of foil, about 12-inches long. Divide sausage, shrimp, spinach, onion, tomatoes and potatoes into 4 equal portions and add to the center of each foil in a single layer.

Fold up all 4 sides of each foil packet.

Sprinkle olive oil and seasoning mix evenly over the top and gently toss to combine. Divide water amongst the four packets, about 2 tablespoons per pack. Fold the sides of the foil over the shrimp, covering completely and sealing the packets closed.

Place foil packets on cooking sheet and bake for about 12-15 minutes. Before opening packets, cut slits into the pack to allow steam to escape. Carefully open, garnish with parsley and serve.

OPTION: Instead of baking, preheat grill and placed closed foil packets directly on rake. Grill on medium low heat for about 15 minutes.

Nutritional information:

Total calories: 229

Vitamins: Vitamin A 178µg, Vitamin B6 0.4mg, Vitamin B12 1.5µg, Vitamin C 26mg, Vitamin K 113µg

Minerals: Phosphorus 365mg, Selenium 54µg, Magnesium 32mg

Sugars 4g

9.   Berry Blue Grilled Chicken Salad

Out of all berries, blueberries are most beneficial. When combined with raspberries and strawberries, such as in this fresh summer salad, the combined nutrients can slow the progression of age-related brain degeneration while improving learning, memory, and motor skills.

Ingredients:

- 1/4 cup apple cider vinegar
- 2 tablespoon honey
- 1/2 cup blueberries
- 1/4 cup olive oil
- 1/4 cup raspberries
- 1/4 cup strawberries, halved
- 1/2 cup pecans, chopped
- 1 cup romaine lettuce, chopped
- 1 cup baby spinach
- 1 cup baby arugula
- 2 cups cooked chicken breast, cubed

How to prepare:

In a blender, combine vinegar, honey, and 1/4 cup blueberries. Blend until smooth, slowly add olive oil until mix is the consistency of salad dressing – set aside.

In a large bowl, combine remaining ingredients. Drizzle with a few tablespoons of blueberry dressing, toss to lightly coat.

Separate into serving bowls, serve with additional dressing if desired.

Nutritional information:

Total calories: 518

Vitamins: Vitamin A 137µg, Vitamin B6 1.3mg, Vitamin C 26mg, Vitamin K 125µg,

Minerals: Niacln 14mg, Phosphorus 420mg, Selenium 46µg, Zinc 3mg

Sugars: 24g

10.   Blackened Salmon with Ginger Bok Choy

Not only is this salmon exploding with spice, it is exploding with Omega 3s and phosphorus. Phosphorus allows healthy brain cells to thrive and remain strong while improving cognitive function.

Ingredients:

- 1 tablespoon dried thyme
- 1 teaspoon garlic powder
- 1 teaspoon onion powder
- 1 tablespoon dried oregano
- 1 tablespoon smoked paprika
- 1 teaspoon red pepper
- Kosher or sea salt to taste
- 1 (6 ounce) salmon fillets
- 2 tablespoon olive oil
- 2 green onion, chopped
- 1 tablespoon ginger root, grated
- 2 cloves garlic, grated
- 2 cups bok choy, chopped
- 1 tablespoon water

- 1/2 lime, juiced

How to prepare:

Combine spices in a small bowl. Coat each side of salmon with spice mix. Allow to rest for 5 to 10 minutes.

Meanwhile, heat 1 tablespoon olive oil in large skillet on medium heat. Once hot, place salmon skin side up. Cook until fish begins to brown and turns crisp. Carefully turn salmon over and continue to cook second side until crisp. Remove from pan and rest.

In separate medium skillet, heat remaining oil. Add green onion, ginger and garlic. Cook, stirring frequently, until mix begins to brown. Add bok choy and water, continue to cook until bok choy is wilted and water is evaporating.

Serve salmon on top of bok choy and drizzled with lime juice.

Nutritional information:

Total calories: 559

Vitamins: Vitamin B6 0.8mg, Vitamin B12µg, Vitamin D 27µg, Vitamin K 57µg

Minerals: Phosphorus 832mg, Selenium 155µg, Niacin 25mg

Sugars: 1g

11. Asian Peanut Chicken Salad

Leafy greens are loaded with Vitamin C, making this Asian inspired entrée salad extra beneficial. The highest levels of Vitamin C are found in the brain and its tissues where brain energy is most frequently used. Allow this salad to regulate the neurochemicals in your brain!

Ingredients:

- 1 lime, juiced
- 2 tablespoons hoisin sauce
- 1 teaspoon honey
- 1 teaspoon ginger root, grated
- 1 clove garlic, grated
- 1/4 cup peanut butter
- 2 tablespoons rice wine vinegar
- 1 teaspoon toasted sesame oil
- 1/4 cup chopped peanuts
- 2 cups cooked chicken breast, cubed
- 1 cup bok choy, chopped
- 1 cup kale, chopped
- 1 cup Napa cabbage, chopped
- 1/2 red bell pepper, thinly sliced

- 1/2 small red onion, thinly sliced

- 2 tablespoons fresh cilantro, chopped

How to prepare:

In blender, combine lime juice, hoisin, honey, ginger, garlic, peanut butter, vinegar, and oil until consistency of salad dressing.

Combine remaining ingredients. Add a few tablespoons of peanut dressing and toss just to coat. Separate into serving bowls, garnish with fresh cilantro.

Nutritional information:

Total calories: 441

Vitamins: Vitamin A 216µg, Vitamin B6 1.2mg, Vitamin C 82mg, Vitamin K 183µg

Minerals: Niacin 14mg, Magnesium 115mg, Phosphorus 397mg, Selenium 32µg

Sugars: 9g

12. Sweet Potato and Black Bean Burrito

Beta-carotene rich sweet potatoes combined with the perfect protein of black beans and brown rice make this burrito a powerhouse of brain nutrients. Not only will the sweet potato boost memory, but your immune system as well. The sweet potato has been used to maintain cognitive development in some of the oldest cultures in the world.

Ingredients:

- 1 sweet potato, peeled and cubed
- 1 tablespoon olive oil
- 1 tablespoon chili powder
- 1 teaspoon ground cumin
- Pinch of Kosher salt
- 4 large whole wheat flour tortillas
- 1/4 cup corn kernels
- 1/2 cup cooked black beans
- 1 cup cooked long grain brown rice
- 1 cup shredded romaine
- 1 yellow pepper, sliced
- 1/2 red onion, sliced
- 1/4 cup salsa

How to prepare:

Preheat oven to 400 degrees

Toss sweet potato in olive oil, chili powder, cumin, and salt. Place on cooking sheet and roast until potatoes are soft and beginning to brown. About 15 to 20 minutes.

Place tortillas on flat surface, divide potatoes and all other ingredients equally between each tortilla. Fold in side and roll to form burrito. Serve.

Nutritional information:

Total calories: 317

Vitamins: Vitamin A 337µg, Vitamin B6 0.3mg, Vitamin C 37mg

Minerals: Phosphorus 207mg, Magnesium 6

Mg, Thiamin 0.4mg

Sugars: 6g

13.   Avocado Pasta

Not only do fresh herbs add flavor to any dish, but they're packed with nutrients! Vitamins E and K, found in fresh herbs, paired with the healthy fat of the avocado make this a well-rounded and filling pasta dish.

Ingredients:

- 2 tablespoons olive oil
- 6 spears asparagus, cut into 1 inch pieces
- 2 cloves garlic, minced
- 1/2 yellow onion, sliced
- 1 cup sweet peas, fresh or frozen (thawed)
- 1 pound cooked whole wheat penne pasta
- 2 tablespoons fresh basil, chopped
- 2 tablespoons fresh rosemary, minced
- 2 tablespoons fresh oregano, chopped
- 1 ripe avocado, cut into 1/2-inch chunks
- 1/2 cup shredded Parmesan cheese

How to prepare:

In medium skillet, heat oil on medium heat. Add asparagus, garlic, and onion. Cook until onion begins to soften and add sweet peas. Add Penne, cook until penne are hot. If the pasta beings to stick to the pan, add a tablespoon of water.

Toss in basil, oregano, avocado, and parmesan. Once parmesan just begins to melt, spoon until serving bowls.

Nutritional information:

Total calories: 589

Vitamins: Vitamin B6 0.5mg, Vitamin E 3mg, Vitamin K 50µg

Minerals: Magnesium 132mg, Phosphorus 433mg, Selenium 85µg, Zinc 4mg

Sugars: 6g

14. Eggplant Lasagna

Filled with Vitamin K, this pasta-free lasagna is a brain booster. Vitamin K regulates the calcium in the brain improving overall brain health.

Ingredients:

- 1 (24 ounce) jar marinara sauce, preferably homemade
- 1 tablespoon olive oil
- 1 medium yellow onion, sliced
- 1 cup mushrooms, minced
- Kosher or sea salt to taste
- 2 cloves garlic, minced
- 3 cups spinach, chopped
- 1 cup ricotta cheese
- 1 1/2 cups shredded mozzarella
- 1/2 cup cottage cheese (small curd if possible)
- 2 egg white
- 1 teaspoon fresh oregano, chopped
- 1 teaspoon fresh basil, chopped
- 1/2 teaspoon black pepper

- 2 large eggplant, sliced 1/4 inch thick lengthwise
- 1/4 cup grated parmesan cheese

How to prepare:

Preheat oven to 425 degrees. Coat a 13" x 9" x 2" casserole dish with non-stick spray and spread 1 1/4 cups of marinara on the bottom of the dish.

In a large skillet, add oil and heat on medium-low. Sauté onion until onions are soft and begin to brown. Add mushrooms, and pinch of salt. Mushrooms will begin to release water, cook until this water evaporates, about 2 to 3 minutes. Add garlic and spinach, sauté until spinach is wilted, about 3 minutes. Remove from heat and cool.

In a large mixing bowl, combine ricotta, 1 cup mozzarella, cottage cheese, egg white, oregano, basil, and pepper.

Arrange sliced eggplant flat in casserole dish add 1/4 cup cheese mix, spread evenly to cover noodles. On top of the cheese, evenly spread 1/4 cup of cooked vegetables. Repeat process until no cheese or vegetable filling is left, ending with eggplant on top. Evenly spread 1 cup marinara over rolls, sprinkle with remaining mozzarella and parmesan.

Cover with aluminum foil and bake 20 minutes, or until cheese is hot and bubbly. If desired, serve with additional heated marinara.

Nutritional information:

Total calories: 315

Vitamins: Vitamin A 210 µg, Vitamin B6 0.5mg, Vitamin B12 0.9 µg, Vitamin K 98µg

Minerals: Calcium 444mg, Potassium 1050mg, Riboflavin 0.5mg, Niacin 6mg

Sugars: 15g

15.   Ahi Tuna Burger with Arugula and Tarragon Yogurt Aioli

A great alternative to salmon, Ahi tuna is packed with B Vitamins. The nutrients found in this fish allow for optimal oxygen circulation, providing the brain with all the resources it needs for ultimate brain function.

Ingredients:

- 1/2-pound ahi tuna, minced
- 2 tablespoons onion, minced
- 1 egg
- 3 cloves garlic, minced and divided
- 2 tablespoons ground pistachios
- 1/4 teaspoon cayenne pepper
- 2 tablespoons lime juice, divided
- 1 tablespoon sesame oil
- 1/2 cup plain Greek yogurt
- 2 tablespoons fresh tarragon, chopped
- 1/4 cup shredded cucumber
- 1/2 cup baby arugula
- 2 whole wheat hamburger buns

How to prepare:

Combine tuna, onion, egg, one clove garlic, cayenne pepper, pistachios, and 1 tablespoon lime juice. Form into patties. Patties will be very fragile.

Heat sesame oil in skillet on medium heat. Once hot, place tuna patties in pan and cook until medium and some pink remains (fish can be cooked well-done if desired).

While cooking, combine remaining lime juice, remaining garlic, Greek yogurt, tarragon. Squeeze excess water from cucumber and add to yogurt mixture.

Spread yogurt sauce on to bun, followed by tuna burger. Top with arugula and top bun. Serve.

Nutritional information:

Total calories: 416

Vitamins: Vitamin B6 1.4mg, Vitamin B12 2.8µg

Minerals: Phosphorus 559mg, Niacin 23mg

Sugars: 7g

16.   Pecan Crusted Salmon with Roasted Brussels Sprouts

The trio of pecans, salmon, and Brussel sprouts make this meal a nutrient rich cornucopia. This dish is well rounded with Vitamins B, C, D, and K and loaded with Omega 3s and Niacin. Niacin slows the rate of cognitive loss, allowing improved memory and antioxidant functions of the brain.

Ingredients:

- 1 pound Brussels sprouts, stems removed cut in half
- 2 tablespoons olive oil, divided
- 1 teaspoon salt, divided
- 1/2 teaspoon black pepper
- 1 clove garlic, minced
- 2 (6 ounces) salmon filets
- 1/2 cup pecans, ground
- 1 teaspoon cayenne pepper

How to prepare:

Preheat oven to 400 degrees. Spray cooking sheet with nonstick spray.

Toss Brussels sprouts with half the olive oil, half the salt, pepper, and garlic. Place on cooking sheet and bake for 15 minutes.

Brush the salmon with remaining olive oil. Combine the pecans, remaining salt, and cayenne. Press the pecan mixture onto the salmon.

Remove Brussels sprouts from oven and turn. Place crusted salmon on pan with Brussels sprouts and return to the oven for an additional 10 to 15 minutes until salmon is flaky and Brussels sprouts are crispy.

Nutritional information:

Total calories: 757

Vitamins: Vitamin B6 0.9mg, Vitamin B12 7.8µg, Vitamin C 82mg, Vitamin D 27µg, Vitamin K 168µg

Minerals: Phosphorus 939mg, Selenium 157µg, Niacin 25mg

Sugars: 3g

17. Slow Cooker Sweet Potato Chili

Quick and easy brain food for a busy day. Sweet potato makes this meatless chili flavorful and filling. Packed with Vitamin A and C it's the perfect balance of delicious and nutritious.

Ingredients:

- 1 large sweet potato, peeled and diced
- 1 large onion, diced
- 1 jalapeno, seeds removed, diced
- 1 teaspoon garlic powder
- 3 tablespoons chili powder
- 1 tablespoon ground cumin
- 1 teaspoon smoked paprika
- 1 1/2 cups water
- 2 cups black beans
- 2 (14-ounce) can diced tomatoes

How to prepare:

Combine all ingredients in slow cooker. Cook on low for 8 hours. Serve.

Nutritional information:

Total calories: 228

Vitamins: Vitamin A 497µg, Vitamin B6 0.6mg, Vitamin C 51mg

Minerals: Phosphorus 231mg, Magnesium 96mg, Thiamin 1.5mg

Sugars: 10g

18. Slow Cooker Coconut Cashew Chicken with Vegetables

Enjoy this Asian flare with a side of essential vitamins and minerals. A large amount of B6 slows shrinkage of the brain and reduces gray matter atrophy in areas most susceptible to memory loss.

Ingredients:

- 3 skinless boneless chicken breasts
- 1 onion, diced
- 1 (14oz) can unsweetened coconut milk
- 1 cup water
- 1/2 cup ground cashews
- 2 tablespoons tomato paste
- 2 clove garlic, minced
- 2 teaspoons hoisin sauce
- 1 teaspoon turmeric
- 1/2 teaspoon curry powder
- 1/2 teaspoon cayenne pepper
- 1 carrot, peeled and diced
- 3 stalks celery, diced
- 4 red potatoes, skin on, cut into quarters

- 2 cups kale, chopped

How to prepare:

Combine all ingredients in slow cooker except for kale. Cook on low for 8 hours or high for 4 hours.

Add kale, allow kale to wilt, about 5 minutes. Serve.

Nutritional information:

Total calories: 570

Vitamins: Vitamin A 314µg, Vitamin B6 1.0mg, Vitamin C 58mg Vitamin K 253µg

Minerals: Magnesium 153mg, Phosphorus 465mg, Selenium 33µg

Sugars: 10g

19. Salmon Salad Sandwich

A light meal option, this salmon salad sandwich contains selenium. Acting as an antioxidant, selenium repairs nerve cells preventing cognitive decline.

Ingredients:

- 8 ounces' salmon, cooked and flaked
- 3 tablespoons plain Greek yogurt
- 2 teaspoons lime juice
- 2 teaspoon fresh tarragon, chopped
- 1 teaspoon dry dill
- 4 slices tomato
- 4 slices red onion
- 1/2 cup baby spinach
- 4 slices whole wheat bread, toasted

How to prepare:

Combine salmon, yogurt, lime, tarragon, and dill. Mix well, taste and add more seasoning if desired.

Divide salmon spread between two slices of wheat bread. Top with tomato, onion, and spinach. Place second slice of bread on top and serve.

Nutritional information:

Total calories: 345

Vitamins: Vitamin B6 0.5mg, Vitamin B12 3.3µg, Vitamin D 11µg, Vitamin K 55µg

Minerals: Phosphorus 493mg, Selenium 78µg, Niacin 13mg

Sugars: 6g

20. Greek Chicken Spinach Salad with Yogurt Dressing

Combine with spinach, walnuts make this a superfood packed salad with Mediterranean flare. Antioxidants protect against degeneration while B vitamins give brain cells energy and new life.

Ingredients:

- 4 clove garlic, minced, divided
- 2 teaspoons dry oregano
- 2 tablespoons lemon juice, divided
- 1 tablespoon olive oil
- 2 skinless boneless chicken breast
- 1/2 cup shredded cucumber
- 1 cup Greek yogurt
- 2 teaspoons dry dill
- 4 cups spinach
- 1/4 cup walnuts
- 1/4 cup feta cheese

How to prepare:

Combine 2 cloves of the garlic, oregano, 1 tablespoon lemon juice and olive oil. Pour over chicken breast. Set aside and marinate for 30 minutes. After marinating, cook in skillet on medium heat until internal temperature reaches 165 and no pink remains. Set aside to rest.

In small bowl, combine cucumber (squeezed of excess water), yogurt, dill, remaining garlic, and remaining lemon juice. Mix well.

In two bowls, divide spinach equally. Add 1 tablespoon yogurt dressing into each bowl and toss just until leaves are coated. Top with walnuts, feta cheese and chicken – serve.

Nutritional information:

Total calories: 452

Vitamins: Vitamin A 319µg, Vitamin B6 1.2mg, Vitamin K 317µg

Minerals: Phosphorus 481mg, Selenium 36µg, Riboflavin 0.5mg, Niacin 10mg

Sugars: 7g

21. Seared Salmon with Spinach and Sundried Tomatoes

This may be the simplest of recipes, packed with flavor and an abundance of vitamins and minerals. With over daily recommendations of Vitamin B12, Vitamin D, and Niacin, this easy recipe will boost your brains cognitive abilities!

Ingredients:

- 2 (8oz) salmon filets
- Salt and pepper to taste
- 1 tablespoon olive oil, divided
- 1 clove garlic, minced
- 1/2 cup sundried tomatoes, chopped
- 2 cups spinach

How to prepare:

Lightly season both sides of salmon with salt and pepper. Heat half the olive oil in skillet on medium heat. Once hot, place salmon skin side down. Cook approximately 6 minutes and flip. Continue to cook until just flaky.

Meanwhile, in a separate skillet, heat remaining oil. Once hot, add garlic and sun dried tomatoes. Cook until fragrant, about 1 to 2 minutes. Add spinach, cook until wilted. Serve on top of salmon.

Nutritional information:

Total calories: 597

Vitamins: Vitamin B6 0.9mg, Vitamin B12 9.6µg, Vitamin D 33µg, Vitamin K 84µg

Minerals: Potassium 1944mg, Phosphorus 1037mg, Selenium 191µg, Niacin 31mg

Sugars: 5g

22.   Berry and Apple Salad with Cider Dressing

This crisp refreshing salad is the perfect light meal of a fall evening. A variety of leafy greens pack this salad with Vitamin K, strengthening brain cells and nerves.

Ingredients:

- 1 tablespoon honey
- 1/4 cup apple juice
- 3 tablespoons apple cider vinegar
- 2 tablespoons olive oil
- 1 cup romaine
- 1/2 cup baby arugula
- 1/2 cup spinach
- 1/2 cup kale
- 1 medium gala apple, sliced thin
- 1/4 cup blackberries
- 1/4 cup blueberries

How to prepare:

Combine honey, juice, vinegar, and oil in blender. Blend until well combine and the consistency of salad dressing.

In large bowl, combine remaining ingredients with 2 to 3

tablespoons of dressing. Lightly toss. Divide into serving bowls. Serve with additional dressing. If desired, chicken or salmon can be added.

Nutritional information:

Total calories: 234

Vitamins: Vitamin C 27mg, Vitamin K 149µg

Minerals: Folate 49µg, Magnesium 26g

Sugars: 22g

23.   Chicken and Apple Spinach Wrap

Celery added to this wrap, or any dish, is a low-calorie option with great brain benefit. While not changing the flavor of any recipe, celery boosts oxygen flow to the brain promoting healthy cells and overall brain function.

Ingredients:

- 1 boneless skinless chicken breast, shredded
- 1 medium apple, cubed
- 2 celery stalk, minced
- 2 tablespoons onion, minced
- 3 tablespoons plain Greek yogurt
- 2 teaspoons honey
- 1/2 cup spinach
- 2 large whole wheat tortillas

How to prepare:

Combine all ingredients except spinach and tortilla.

Lay tortillas on flat surface. Divide spinach between both tortillas, top with chicken mixture. Fold in side of tortilla and roll to form burrito shape. Serve.

Nutritional information:

Total calories: 256

Vitamins: Vitamin B6 0.6mg, Vitamin K 44µg

Minerals: Phosphorus 260mg, Selenium 28µg, Niacin 6mg

Sugars: 15g

24. Blackened Ahi Tuna with Mango Salsa and Avocado

Take a break from salmon and kick Vitamin B into high gear with Ahi Tuna! A great alternative to salmon, Ahi tuna contains enough Vitamin B to give you extra energy and improve concentration.

Ingredients:

- 1 teaspoon cayenne pepper
- 1/2 teaspoon garlic powder
- 1/2 teaspoon onion powder
- 1/4 teaspoon Kosher salt
- 1/2 teaspoon black pepper
- 1 teaspoon paprika
- 1 teaspoon chili powder
- 1 tablespoon olive oil
- 2 (6oz) Ahi Tuna Filets
- 1 large tomato, diced
- 1 small red onion, diced
- 1/4 cup mango, diced
- 1 tablespoon lime juice
- 2 teaspoon fresh cilantro, chopped

- 1 tablespoon jalapeno pepper, minced

How to prepare:

Combine cayenne, garlic powder, onion powder, salt, pepper, paprika, and chili powder. Brush tuna filets with olive oil and season well with spice mix.

Heat skillet on medium heat, place tuna in pan and cook until the first side begins to brown. Flip, and continue cooking on second side, about 3 minutes. Tuna should still be pink on the inside.

In medium bowl, combine remaining ingredients. Allow to rest for about 5 minutes. Spoon on top of cooked tuna. Serve.

Nutritional information:

Total calories: 370

Vitamins: Vitamin B6 2.4mg, Vitamin B12 4.7µg

Minerals: Phosphorus 682mg, Selenium 207µg, Niacin 43mg

Sugars: 7g

25.   Peanut Chicken Lettuce Wraps

An entrée or an appetizer, this carb free favorite is loaded with Vitamin K. A key anti-aging component, Vitamin K keeps the mind sharp. By proving and regulating calcium to brain cells, Vitamin K keeps the brain functioning.

Ingredients:

- 1 pound ground chicken
- 1 tablespoon sesame oil
- 2 cloves garlic, minced
- 1 yellow onion, diced
- 2 tablespoons creamy peanut butter
- 1 tablespoon honey
- 2 tablespoons rice vinegar
- 2 tablespoons hoisin
- 1 head bib lettuce
- 1/2 cup shredded carrots
- 1/2 cup cucumber, diced small
- 1/2 cup red bell pepper, diced small
- 1/4 cup sliced green onions
- 3 tablespoons fresh cilantro, chopped

How to prepare:

In skillet, cook ground chicken until no pink remains. Drain off any excess liquid. Set aside.

In small sauce pan, heat sesame oil. Add garlic and onion. Cook until garlic is fragrant and onion is soft. Add peanut butter, honey, vinegar, and hoisin sauce. Whisk until smooth. Bring to a boil, reduce heat and simmer for 2 minutes. Gradually add to cooked ground chicken, just until all chicken is coated.

Carefully remove and separate leaves from head of bib lettuce. On each leave, spoon about 2 tablespoons chicken and top with carrot, cucumber, pepper, onion, and cilantro. Serve.

Nutritional information:

Total calories: 299

Vitamins: Vitamin A 237µg, Vitamin B6, 0.6mg, Vitamin C 31mg, Vitamin K 63µg

Minerals: Riboflavin 0.3mg, Niacin 7mg

Sugars: 11g

26.   Seared Steak with Baked Tomatoes and Spinach

Strictly found in meat, this succulent steak recipe contains carnosine, which is a little known but powerful nutrient. Carnosine is created from two amino acid is found in muscles and brain tissues. Maintaining carnosine is important in preventing degenerative processes in the brain and prevents premature aging.

Ingredients:

- 2 large tomatoes
- 2 tablespoons olive oil, divided
- 2 clove garlic, minced and divided
- 1/2 teaspoon ground turmeric
- 1/2 teaspoon ground cumin
- 1/2 teaspoon chili powder
- 1 teaspoon paprika
- 1/4 teaspoon black pepper
- 2 (6oz) Sirloin steaks
- 1/2 teaspoon salt
- 3 cups spinach

How to prepare:

Preheat oven to 400 degrees. Coat tomatoes with 1 tablespoon of olive oil and half the garlic. Bake for 15-20 minutes, or until soft

Combine turmeric, cumin, chili powder, paprika, and black pepper. Coat steaks on each side with spice mix

In medium skillet, heat 1 tablespoon olive oil. On medium heat, cook steaks until medium. A little pink in the middle or internal temperature of 150 degrees.

Remove steak from pan to rest. In the same skillet, the steaks were cooked in, add spinach and remaining garlic. Cook on medium heat until wilted. Serve with steak and baked tomato.

Nutritional information:

Total calories: 346

Vitamins: Vitamin A 195µg, Vitamin B6 0.9mg, B12 1.6µg, Vitamin K 161µg

Minerals: Phosphorus 317mg, Selenium 43µg, Zinc 7mg

Sugars: 2g

27. Salmon Cakes with Bok Choy and Wasabi Lime Aioli

Typically over looked, Wasabi is a great way to and a punch and nutrients to a recipe! Wasabi contains many vitamins and minerals and is known to help with inflammation.

Ingredients:

- 2 (6oz) salmon filets, minced
- 3 egg whites
- 2 teaspoons dry dill
- 2 green onion, diced
- 1 tablespoon lemon juice
- 3 tablespoons whole wheat Panko bread crumbs
- 1/2 teaspoon Kosher salt
- 2 tablespoons olive oil, divided
- 1 tablespoon grated ginger
- 2 clove garlic, grated and divided
- 3 cups bok choy
- 3 tablespoons mayonnaise
- 3 tablespoons lime juice
- 1 teaspoon wasabi paste (more if desired)
- Water, as needed

How to prepare:

Combine salmon, egg, dill green onion, lemon juice, Panko and salt. Mix well and form into patties.

In medium skillet, heat half the olive oil. On medium heat, cook the salmon patties until brown. Flip and continue to cook until done throughout.

Meanwhile, heat the remaining olive oil. On medium heat, add half the garlic and ginger. Cook until garlic just begins to brown. Add bok choy and cook until wilted.

In a small bowl combine mayonnaise, lime juice, wasabi past, and remaining garlic. Mix well. If needed, add water to make aioli the consistency of salad dressing.

Serve salmon cakes on top of bok choy. Drizzle with wasabi lime aioli.

Nutritional information:

Total calories: 626

Vitamins: Vitamin A 346µg, Vitamin B6 1.3mg, Vitamin B12 8.3µg, Vitamin C 70mg, Vitamin D 19µg, Vitamin K 122µg

Minerals: Phosphorus 557µg, Selenium 67µg, Niacin 16mg

Sugars: 5g

28.   Slow Cooker White Bean Chicken Soup

A great alternative to the black or kidney beans, cannellini beans are just as beneficial. Adding a more buttery flavor and texture, this bean is very versatile in great in light soups, chilies and stews. This little bean improves cognitive ability and detoxifies.

Ingredients:

- 1 teaspoon fresh sage, chopped
- 1 teaspoon fresh rosemary, chopped
- 1 pound skinless boneless chicken breasts, cut into 1-inch pieces
- 1 small onion, diced
- 2 medium carrots, peeled and diced
- 2 large celery stalks, diced
- 2 large tomatoes, diced
- 3 tablespoons tomato paste
- 3 cups chicken bone broth
- 1 cup water
- 2 cups cannellini beans
- 2 cups kale, chopped

How to prepare:

Combine all ingredients, except for kale, in slow cooker. Cook on high for 4 hours or low for 8 hours. Before serving, stir in kale and cook just until wilted. Ladle into serving bowls.

Nutritional information:

Total calories: 313

Vitamins: Vitamin A 210µg, Vitamin B6 0.8mg, Vitamin C 65mg, Vitamin K 254µg

Minerals: Phosphorus 373mg, Selenium 25µg, Niacin 13mg

Sugars: 4g

29.   Shrimp Stuffed Avocado

Shrimp and avocado are a great pair, not only in recipes but in creating a meal well balanced in important vitamins and minerals. Both contain healthy fats and cholesterol to improve brain function, blood flow, and healthy brain cells and nerves. All of which work together to prevent cognitive degeneration.

Ingredients:

- 2 avocados

- 2 cups cooked shrimp, diced

- 1 celery stalk, minced

- 2 tablespoons onion, minced

- 2 teaspoon dry dill

- 1/4 cup plain Greek yogurt

- 1 tablespoon mayonnaise

- 1 teaspoon lemon juice

How to prepare:

Cut avocados in half, remove pit and scoop out a bit of the center to create a boat. Place scooped out avocado in medium mixing bowl. Skin can be left on, or removed if desired.

Mash the scooped out avocado. Combine remaining ingredients with mashed avocado. Spoon into avocado boats. Serve.

Nutritional information:

Total calories: 423

Vitamins: Vitamin B6 0.7mg, Vitamin B12 1.4µg, Vitamin K 57µg

Minerals: Phosphorus 428mg, Selenium 56µg

Sugars: 3g

30.   Warm Chickpea Salad

While typically used for hummus, the chickpea is a very versatile bean. In this warm salad, the chickpea adds a post of protein while boosting memory. This salad is a great meal for improving the quality of sleep, which the brain needs to regenerate each day.

Ingredients:

- 1 tablespoon olive oil
- 1 small red onion, diced
- 1 small red bell pepper, diced
- 2 clove garlic, minced
- 1 medium tomato, diced
- 2 cups chickpeas
- 2 cups Spinach
- 2 tablespoon fresh basil, chopped
- 1/2 cup shredded parmesan cheese
- 1 tablespoon lemon juice

How to prepare:

Heat olive oil in skillet over medium heat. Once hot, add onion, bell pepper, and garlic. Cook until onions are soft. Add tomato, spinach and chickpeas. Cook until spinach is wilted and chickpeas are hot. Stir in basil and parmesan until cheese is melted. Spoon into serving plates and drizzle lemon juice on top and serve.

Nutritional information:

Total calories: 316

Vitamins: Vitamin K 115μg

Minerals: Phosphorus 293mg, Folate 159μg

Sugars: 8g

31. Taco Stuffed Bell Pepper

A great low carb alternative to a traditional taco! The blend of black beans and brown rice not only combine to make a perfect protein, but make this little pepper a filling meal.

Ingredients:

- 2 large red bell peppers
- 1 tablespoon olive oil, divided
- 1 clove garlic, minced
- 1 small onion, chopped
- 1 cup black beans, cooked
- 1 cup cooked brown rice
- 2 cups salsa, preferably homemade
- 1/4 cup fresh cilantro, chopped
- 1/4 cup shredded cheddar cheese

How to prepare:

Preheat oven to 375 degrees.

Cut off the tops of the peppers, carefully scoop out the seeds and white ribs creating a bowl. Place on cooking sheet sprayed with nonstick spray.

Heat olive oil in large sauté pan over medium heat and add onions and garlic. Mix in beans, rice, and salsa. Cook until warmed through.

Spoon mixture into peppers and top with cheese. Bake 20 to 25 minutes, until peppers are soft and filling is hot.

Nutritional information:

Total calories: 536

Vitamins: Vitamin A 325µg, Vitamin B6 1.1mg, Vitamin C 261mg, Vitamin E 8mg, Vitamin K 44µg

Minerals: Magnesium 138mg, Phosphorus 387mg, Folate 180µg, Thiamin 0.5mg

Sugars: 15g

32. Spiced Meatballs with Tomato Brown Rice

Everyone loves a good meatball. Venture out from the norm with this spiced meatball. Containing turmeric, a little-known spice, makes this meatball a powerful anti-inflammatory agent. In addition, turmeric is a strong antioxidant and has shown to improve the regeneration of cells in the brain stem.

Ingredients:

- 1 cup whole wheat Panko bread crumbs
- 1 pound extra lean ground beef
- 2 egg whites
- 1 small onion, diced and divided
- 4 cloves garlic, minced and divided
- 1 teaspoon turmeric
- 2 teaspoons paprika
- ¼ teaspoon cayenne
- ½ teaspoon ground cumin
- 2 tablespoons fresh parsley, chopped
- 2 tablespoons fresh cilantro, chopped
- 1 tablespoon olive oil
- 2 cups brown rice, cooked

- 1 (14 ounce) can diced tomatoes

How to prepare:

Preheat oven to 400. Spray cooking sheet with nonstick spray. In large bowl, combine panko, ground beef, egg whites, half the onion, half the garlic, turmeric, paprika, cayenne, cumin, parsley and cilantro. Mix well and roll into one inch balls. Place on cooking sheet and bake 15 to 20 minutes.

In skillet, heat olive oil on medium heat. Add remaining onion and garlic and cook until onions are soft. Add rice and tomatoes. Cook until hot. Serve meatballs on top of rice.

Nutritional Information:

Total calories: 551

Vitamins: Vitamin A 81µg, Vitamin B6 0.9mg, Vitamin B12 3.3µg, Vitamin C 24mg, Vitamin K 56µg

Minerals: Phosphorus 442mg, Selenium 49µg, Zinc 8mg, Riboflavin 1.6mg, Niacin 12mg

Sugars: 8g

33.   Herb Shrimp with Couscous

Shrimp is typically thought of as a source of healthy fat and cholesterol. However, shrimp is one of the most well rounded foods. In addition, shrimp is high is antioxidants and minerals. This allows a small amount of shrimp to go a long way in brain and body health.

Ingredients:

- 2 tablespoons olive oil
- 1 red bell pepper, diced
- 1/2-pound asparagus, cut into 1 inch pieces
- 1 small onion, diced and divided
- 4 clove garlic, minced and divided
- 1 pound raw shrimp, peeled and deveined
- 2 tablespoons lemon juice
- 1 tablespoon fresh basil, chopped
- 2 teaspoons fresh oregano, chopped
- 2 teaspoons fresh rosemary, chopped
- 2 cups couscous, cooked

How to prepare:

Over medium heat, heat half the olive oil in skillet. Add red pepper, asparagus, half the onion, and half the garlic. Cook until veggies begin to soften. Add shrimp and cook until shrimp is pink and firm. Stir in lemon juice, basil, oregano, and rosemary.

In separate skillet, heat remaining oil. Add remaining onion and garlic. Cook until soft. Add couscous, mix well. Heat until hot. Serve shrimp over couscous.

Nutritional information:

Total calories: 749

Vitamins: Vitamin B6 1.8mg, Vitamin B12 2.2µg, Vitamin C 89mg, Vitamin E 9mg, Vitamin K 71µg

Minerals: Magnesium 97mg, phosphorus 535mg, Selenium 141µg Zinc 4mg

Sugars: 6g

34.   Roasted Beet Salad with Orange and Walnuts

Sweet honey and orange citrus make this beet salad a wonderful earthy salad. Beets contain a high level of nitrates, which widen blood vessels and allow an increased blood flow to the brain. A healthy blood flow allows deeper concentration and higher memory capabilities.

Ingredients:

- 2 red beets, peeled and diced large
- 2 golden beets, peeled and diced large
- 2 tablespoons olive oil
- 1 tablespoon fresh rosemary, chopped
- 1 tablespoon orange zest
- 3 cups spinach
- 1 large orange, peeled and cut into wedges
- 1/4 cup walnuts
- 1/4 cup crumbled soft goat cheese
- 2 tablespoons honey
- 2 tablespoons balsamic vinegar

How to prepare:

Preheat oven to 450 degrees.

Toss both beets in olive oil, rosemary, and orange zest. Bake for 20 to 25 minutes, stirring every 10 minutes. Bake until soft. Remove from oven and cool completely.

In large bowl, toss cooked beets, spinach, oranges, walnuts and cheese. Divide into serving bowls. Drizzle with honey and vinegar to serve.

Nutritional information:

Total calories: 473

Vitamins: Vitamin A 292µg, Vitamin C 56mg, Vitamin K 238µg

Minerals: Magnesium 114mg, Phosphorus 232mg

Sugars: 38g

35. Balsamic Veggie Wrap

Balsamic vinegar gives this veggie wrap a little zip to create a wonderful light and quick meal. Packed with several different vegetables, this wrap contains a variety of vitamin and minerals to help with everyday brain function. Keeping the brain alert and energized.

Ingredients:

- 1 tablespoon olive oil
- 1 small zucchini, cut into thin strips
- 1 red bell pepper, cut into thin strips
- 1 small onion, cut into thin strips
- 1/4 cup mushrooms, chopped
- 1/2 cup spinach
- 2 clove garlic, minced
- 2 tablespoon honey
- 1/4 cup balsamic vinegar
- 2 large whole wheat tortillas

How to prepare:

In medium skillet, heat olive oil on medium heat. Once hot, combine all ingredients with exception of honey, vinegar, and tortillas. Cook until veggies are soft.

In small sauce pan, combine honey and vinegar. Cook on medium heat, bring to a boil and simmer until slightly thickened. Stir frequently.

On flat surface, lay tortillas. Divide cooked veggies between the tortillas and drizzle vinegar and honey sauce over the top. Fold in the sides and roll into a burrito shape. Serve.

Nutritional information:

Total calories: 522

Vitamins: Vitamin A 284µg, Vitamin B6 0.6mg, Vitamin C 99mg, Vitamin K 190µg

Minerals: Potassium 1047mg, Phosphorus 283mg

Sugars: 44g

umentin

36.   Mediterranean Shrimp with Pasta

A spin on the popular Mediterranean diet, this shrimp pasta dish is a fresh dish overflowing with flavor. Popular Mediterranean spices, such as garlic and capers, provide extra nutrients to improve cognitive function and decrease the decline of brain activity.

Ingredients:

- 1 tablespoon olive oil
- 1/2-pound raw shrimp, peeled and deveined
- 2 clove garlic, minced
- 1 small onion, diced
- 1/4 cup zucchini, diced
- 1/4 cup eggplant, diced
- 1/4 cup capers, drained and dried
- 1 cup spinach
- 1/2 cup tomatoes, diced
- 4 cups whole grain pasta, cooked
- 1/4 cup shredded parmesan

How to prepare:

In skillet, heat oil to medium heat. Add shrimp, garlic, onion, zucchini, and eggplant. Cook until shrimp just begins to firm and veggies are soft. Add capers, spinach, and tomato. Cook until spinach is wilted and tomatoes are hot. Toss in pasta, continue to simmer until pasta is heated through. Top with shredded parmesan

Nutritional information:

Total calories: 517

Vitamins: Vitamin A 184 µg, Vitamin B6 0.5mg, Vitamin B12 1.6µg, Vitamin K 88µg

Minerals: Calcium 360mg, Magnesium 132mg, Phosphorus 598mg, Selenium 97µg, Zink 4mg

Sugars: 5g

37.   Paprika Chicken with Beans and Quinoa

This well-rounded chicken entrée is a great source of iron. Iron is directly connected to brain health and functions. Not only does iron assist in proper blood flow, it creates neural pathways to help with the prevention of cognitive decline.

Ingredients:

- 1 tablespoon olive oil
- 2 boneless skinless chicken breast, cut into cubes
- 2 tablespoons Paprika
- 2 clove garlic, minced
- 2 cups fresh green beans, trimmed
- 1 cup butter beans
- 1/2 cup cashews
- 2 cups quinoa, cooked

How to prepare:

Add olive oil to skillet and heat on medium. Add chicken and cook until no pink remains. Mix in paprika, garlic and green beans. Continue to cook until beans just begin to soften. Stir in butter beans and cashews. Serve alongside cooked quinoa.

Nutritional information:

Total calories: 714

Vitamins: Vitamin A 199µg, Vitamin B6 1.1mg, Vitamin B12 1µg, Vitamin K 63µg

Minerals: Iron 8mg, Magnesium 247mg, Phosphorus 803mg, and Selenium 77mg, Zinc 6mg

Sugars: 7g

38. Spinach and Pesto Fettuccini with Sundried Tomatoes

A little used ingredient, sundried tomatoes contain higher amounts of Vitamin C and A than raw tomatoes. Both vitamins C and A protect brain cells from free radical damage and are and excellent way to improve overall brain health.

Ingredients:

- 1 tablespoon olive oil
- 2 clove garlic, minced
- 1 cup sundried tomatoes
- 2 cups spinach
- 1/2-pound whole wheat fettuccini, cooked
- 2 tablespoons basil pesto
- 1/4 cup shredded parmesan

How to prepare:

Heat olive oil over medium temperature. Add garlic and sundried tomatoes. Cook until fragrant, add spinach and continue cooking until wilted. Add fettuccini and pesto. Toss to coat in pesto, heat until hot. Divide onto serving dishes, top with parmesan.

Nutritional information:

Total calories: 464

Vitamins: Vitamin A 187µg, Vitamin C 21mg, Vitamin K 178 µg

Minerals: Magnesium 139mg, Phosphorus 365mg, Selenium 47µg, Zinc 3mg

Sugars: 12g

JUICES

1.   Green Watermelon Ginger Juice

Ingredients:

1 cup of watermelon, diced

¼ tsp of ginger, ground

2 cups of Swiss chard, chopped

1 cup of pineapple, chunked

Preparation:

Cut the top of the watermelon. Cut lengthwise in half and then cut one large wedge. Peel it and cut into small cubes. Remove the seeds and fill the measuring cup. Wrap the rest in a plastic foil and refrigerate for later.

Wash the Swiss chard thoroughly under cold running water. Slightly drain and chop into small pieces. Set aside.

Cut the top of the pineapple and peel it using a sharp paring knife. Peel it all and cut into small pieces. Fill the measuring cup and set aside.

Now, combine watermelon, Swiss chard, and pineapple in

a juicer and process until juiced. Transfer to a serving glass and stir in the ginger.

Add some ice and serve immediately.

Enjoy!

Nutrition information per serving: Kcal: 127, Protein: 3.1g, Carbs: 35.8g, Fats: 0.6g

2.   Blueberry Lime Juice

Ingredients:

1 cup of blueberries

1 whole lime, peeled

1 cup of pomegranate seeds

1 small Granny Smith's apple, cored

¼ tsp of ginger, ground

2 oz of water

Preparation:

Place the blueberries in a colander. Rinse well under cold running water and drain. Set aside.

Peel the lime and cut lengthwise in half. Set aside.

Cut the top of the pomegranate fruit using a sharp paring knife. Slice down to each of the white membranes inside of the fruit. Pop the seeds into a measuring cup and set aside.

Wash the apple and cut lengthwise in half. Remove the core and cut into bite-sized pieces and set aside.

Now, combine blueberries, lime, pomegranate seeds, and apple in a juicer and process until juiced. Transfer to a serving glass and stir in the ginger and water.

Refrigerate for 5 minutes before serving.

Enjoy!

Nutritional information per serving: Kcal: 206, Protein: 3.3g, Carbs: 61.1g, Fats: 1.8g

3.   Brussels Sprout Leek Juice

Ingredients:

1 cup of Brussels sprouts

2 large leeks

½ tsp of fresh rosemary

1 large fennel bulb

Preparation:

Wash the Brussels sprouts and trim off the outer leaves. Cut into small pieces and set aside.

Wash the leeks and chop into small pieces. Set aside.

Wash the fennel bulb and trim off the wilted outer layers. Cut into small chunks and set aside.

Now, process Brussels sprouts, fennel, and leeks in a juicer. Transfer to serving glasses and sprinkle with finely chopped rosemary. You can add a dash of Himalayan salt to taste, but this is optional.

Enjoy!

Nutritional information per serving: Kcal: 165, Protein: 8.5g, Carbs: 50.1g, Fats: 1.3g

4.   Carrot Fennel Juice

Ingredients:

1 large carrot, sliced

1 cup of fennel, trimmed and chopped

1 cup of cauliflower, chopped

1 cup of parsnip, sliced

1 whole lime, peeled

Preparation:

Wash and peel the carrot and parsnip. Cut into thin slices and fill the measuring cups. Reserve the rest for later.

Trim off the fennel stalks and outer wilted layers. Wash and chop the fennel into bite-sized pieces. Fill the measuring cup and reserve the rest for later. Set aside.

Wash the cauliflower and trim off the outer leaves. Cut into small pieces and fill the measuring cup. Reserve the rest for later.

Peel the lime and cut lengthwise in half. Set aside.

Now, combine cauliflower, parsnip, carrot, fennel, and lime in a juicer. Process until well juiced.

Transfer to a serving glass and refrigerate for 5 minutes before serving.

Add some turmeric or ginger for some extra taste. However, it's optional.

Nutrition information per serving: Kcal: 141, Protein: 5.6g, Carbs: 46.2g, Fats: 1.1g

5.   Beet Lettuce Juice

Ingredients:

1 cup of beets, chopped

1 cup of red leaf lettuce, shredded

2 large tomatoes, peeled

1 cup of fennel, sliced

1 tbsp of fresh mint, chopped

½ tsp of ginger, ground

Preparation:

Wash the beets and trim off the green ends. Cut into small pieces and set aside.

Wash the lettuce thoroughly and torn with hands. Set aside.

Wash the tomatoes and place them in a bowl. Cut into quarters and reserve the juice while cutting.

Wash the fennel bulb and trim off the wilted outer layers. Cut into small chunks and set aside.

Now, combine beets, lettuce, tomatoes, fennel, and mint in a juicer and process until juiced.

Transfer to serving glasses and stir in the ginger.

Refrigerate for 15 minutes before serving.

Nutritional information per serving: Kcal: 111, Protein: 6.9g, Carbs: 34.8g, Fats: 1.2g

6.   Pumpkin Cucumber Juice

Ingredients:

1 cup of pumpkin, chopped

1 cup of cucumber, sliced

1 cup of butternut squash, cubed

¼ tsp of turmeric, ground

¼ tsp of salt

2 tbsp of water

Preparation:

Peel the pumpkin and cut lengthwise in half. Scoop out the seeds and cut into small cubes. Fill the measuring cup and reserve the rest in the refrigerator.

Wash the cucumber and cut into thin slices. Fill the measuring cup and reserve the rest in the refrigerator.

Cut the squash lengthwise in half. Using a teaspoon, scoop out the seeds and clean it inside. Peel and cut into small cubes. Fill the measuring cup and wrap the rest in a plastic foil and refrigerate.

Now, combine pumpkin, squash, and cucumber in a juicer

and process until juiced. Transfer to a serving glass and stir in the turmeric, salt, and water.

Refrigerate for 5 minutes before serving.

Nutrition information per serving: Kcal: 73, Protein: 4.1g, Carbs: 19.3g, Fats: 0.9g

7. Cilantro Basil Juice

Ingredients:

1 cup of cilantro, chopped

1 cup of fresh basil, torn

1 cup of cucumber, sliced

1 whole lime, peeled

1 medium-sized apple, cored

Preparation:

Wash the cilantro and torn into small pieces. Set aside.

Wash the basil thoroughly under cold running water. Drain and torn into small pieces. Set aside.

Wash the cucumber and cut into thin slices. Fill the measuring cup and reserve the rest for later. Set aside.

Peel the lime and cut lengthwise in half. Set aside.

Wash the apple and cut lengthwise in half. Remove the core and cut into bite-sized pieces. Set aside.

Now, combine cilantro, basil, cucumber, lime, and apple in a juicer and process until well juiced. Transfer to a serving glass and add some crushed ice.

Serve immediately.

Nutritional information per serving: Kcal: 109, Protein: 2.7g, Carbs: 31.9g, Fats: 0.7g

8.   Spinach Fennel Juice

Ingredients:

1 cup of spinach, torn

1 cup of fennel, trimmed and chopped

2 large red bell peppers, seeds removed

1cup of cucumber, sliced

¼ tsp of salt

¼ tsp of cayenne pepper, ground

Preparation:

Rinse the spinach thoroughly under cold running water. Drain and torn into small pieces. Fill the measuring cup and reserve the rest in the refrigerator.

Trim off the fennel stalks and outer wilted layers. Wash and chop the fennel into bite-sized pieces. Fill the measuring cup and reserve the rest for later. Set aside.

Wash the bell peppers and cut each lengthwise in half. Remove the stem and seeds. Chop into small pieces and set aside.

Wash the cucumber and cut into thin slices. Fill the

measuring cup and reserve the rest for later.

Now, combine bell peppers, fennel, spinach, and cucumber in a juicer and process until juiced. Transfer to a serving glass and stir in the salt and cayenne pepper.

Serve cold.

Nutrition information per serving: Kcal: 125, Protein: 10.6g, Carbs: 35.65g, Fats: 2.1g

9.   Broccoli Cabbage Juice

Ingredients:

1 cup of broccoli, chopped

1 cup of green cabbage

1 large cucumber

1 large lemon, peeled

1 tsp liquid honey

Preparation:

Wash the broccoli and trim off the outer wilted layers. Chop into small pieces and fill the measuring cup. Reserve the rest for later.

Wash the cabbage and spinach thoroughly and torn with hands. Set aside.

Wash the cucumber and cut into thick slices. Set aside.

Peel the lemon and cut lengthwise in half. Set aside.

Now, combine broccoli, cabbage, cucumber, and lemon in a juicer and process until well juiced.

Transfer to serving glasses and stir in the honey. Add some ice before serving.

Enjoy!

Nutritional information per serving: Kcal: 150, Protein: 8.8g, Carbs: 36.4g, Fats: 0.9g

10. Swiss Chard Carrot Juice

Ingredients:

1 cup of Swiss chard, torn

1 large carrot, peeled and sliced

1 large wedge of honeydew melon, peeled and cubed

1 cup of cucumber, sliced

1 small ginger knob, peeled

¼ tsp of turmeric, ground

2 oz of water

Preparation:

Rinse the Swiss chard thoroughly under cold running water. Drain and torn into small pieces. Set aside.

Wash and peel the carrot. Cut into thin slices and set aside.

Cut melon lengthwise in half. Scoop out the seeds and then wash. Cut one large wedge and peel it. Cut into small cubes and set aside.

Wash the cucumber and cut into thin slices. Fill the measuring cup and reserve the rest for later. Set aside.

Peel the ginger knob and cut into small pieces. Set aside.

Now, combine Swiss chard, carrot, melon, and cucumber in a juicer and process until juiced. Transfer to a serving glass and stir in the turmeric and water.

Refrigerate for 5 minutes before serving.

Nutrition information per serving: Kcal: 92, Protein: 2.6g, Carbs: 25.7g, Fats: 0.5g

11.　Spicy Lemon Apple Juice

Ingredients:

1 whole lemon, peeled

1 small Golden Delicious apple, cored

1 large carrot, sliced

1 cup of celery, chopped

¼ tsp turmeric, ground

¼ tsp ginger, ground

Preparation:

Peel the lemon and cut lengthwise in half. Set aside.

Wash the apple and cut in half. Remove the core and cut into bite-sized pieces. Set aside.

Wash and peel the carrot. Cut into small slices and set aside.

Wash the celery and cut into small pieces. Set aside.

Now, combine lemon, apple, carrot, and celery in a juicer and process until juiced. Transfer to a serving glass and stir in the water, turmeric, and ginger. If you like, add some crushed ice.

Serve immediately.

Nutrition information per serving: Kcal: 105, Protein: 2.4g, Carbs: 32.8g, Fats: 0.7g

12.   Orange Pomegranate Juice

Ingredients:

1 large orange, peeled

1 cup of pomegranate seeds

1 cup of watermelon, peeled and seeded

1 cup of Romaine lettuce, shredded

Preparation:

Peel the orange and divide into wedges. Set aside.

Cut the top of the pomegranate fruit using a sharp knife. Slice down to each of the white membranes inside of the fruit. Pop the seeds into a medium bowl.

Cut the watermelon lengthwise. For one cup, you will need about 1 large wedge. Peel and cut into chunks. Remove the seeds and set aside.

Wash the lettuce thoroughly. Roughly chop it using hands and add set aside.

Now, process orange, pomegranate seeds, watermelon, and lettuce in a juicer. Transfer to serving glasses and refrigerate before use.

Nutritional information per serving: Kcal: 142, Protein: 5.2g, Carbs: 44.8g, Fats: 1.5g

13. Avocado Peach Juice

Ingredients:

1 cup of avocado, cubed

1 large peach, chopped

1 cup of strawberries, chopped

1 large Granny Smith's apple, cored

¼ tsp of cinnamon, ground

¼ tsp of ginger, ground

2 tsp of coconut water

Preparation:

Peel the avocado and cut in half. Remove the pit and cut into small cubes. Fill the measuring cup and reserve the rest for later.

Wash the peach and cut lengthwise in half. Remove the pit and cut into bite-sized pieces. Set aside.

Wash the strawberries and remove the stems. Cut into bite-sized pieces and fill the measuring cup. Reserve the rest for later.

Wash the apple and cut in half. Remove the core and chop into small pieces. Set aside.

Now, combine avocado, peach, strawberries, and apple in a juicer and process until juiced. Transfer to a serving glass and stir in the cinnamon, ginger, and coconut water.

Refrigerate for 15 minutes before serving.

Nutritional information per serving: Kcal: 386, Protein: 6.5g, Carbs: 68.6g, Fats: 23.2g

14. Asparagus Collard Green Juice

Ingredients:

1 cup of asparagus, trimmed and chopped

1 cup of collard greens, torn

1 medium-sized tomato, chopped

1 cup of spinach, torn

¼ tsp salt

1 rosemary sprig

Preparation:

Wash the asparagus and trim off the woody ends. Cut into small pieces and fill the measuring cup. Set aside.

Combine collard greens and spinach in a large colander. Wash under cold running water and drain. Torn into small pieces and set aside.

Wash the tomato and place it in a small bowl. Cut into small pieces and reserve the tomato juice while cutting. Set aside.

Now, combine asparagus, collard greens, tomato, and spinach in a juicer and process until juiced. Transfer to a serving glass and stir in the reserve tomato juice and salt. Sprinkle with rosemary.

Serve immediately.

Nutritional information per serving: Kcal: 66, Protein: 11.2g, Carbs: 19.6g, Fats: 1.5g

15. Cucumber Lemon Juice

Ingredients:

1 large cucumber, sliced

1 large lemon, peeled

1 cup of avocado, pitted and chopped

1 cup of fresh spinach, torn

1 large lime, peeled

1 small ginger knob, peeled

3 oz of water

Preparation:

Wash the cucumber and cut into thick slices. Set aside.

Peel the lemon and lime. Cut lengthwise in half and set aside.

Peel the avocado and cut in half. Remove the pit and chop into chunks. Set aside.

Wash the spinach thoroughly and torn with hands. Set aside.

Peel the ginger knob and set aside.

Now, combine avocado, cucumber, lemon, lime, spinach, and ginger in a juicer. Process until juiced and transfer to serving glasses. Stir in the water and refrigerate for 20 minutes before serving.

Enjoy!

Nutritional information per serving: Kcal: 269, Protein: 6.7g, Carbs: 35g, Fats: 22.6g

16.   Apple Asparagus Juice

Ingredients:

1 large green apple, cored

1 cup of fresh asparagus, trimmed

3 large oranges, peeled

¼ tsp of turmeric, ground

2 oz of water

Preparation:

Wash the apple and remove the core. Cut into bite-sized pieces and set aside.

Wash the asparagus thoroughly under cold running water and trim off the woody ends. Cut into small pieces and set aside.

Peel the oranges and divide into wedges. Set aside.

Now, combine apple, asparagus, and oranges in a juicer and process until juiced. Transfer to serving glasses and stir in the turmeric and water.

Refrigerate for 10 minutes before serving.

Nutritional information per serving: Kcal: 316, Protein: 9.1g, Carbs: 98.1g, Fats: 1.2g

17.   Watermelon Banana Juice

Ingredients:

1 large wedge of watermelon

1 large banana, sliced

1 cup of strawberries, chopped

2 whole plums, pitted

Preparation:

Cut the watermelon in half. Cut one large wedge and wrap the rest in a plastic foil and refrigerate. Peel the slice and cut into small cubes. Remove the pits and fill the measuring cup. Set aside.

Peel the banana and cut into thin slices. Set aside.

Wash the strawberries and remove the stems. Cut into small pieces and fill the measuring cup. Reserve the rest for in the refrigerator.

Wash the plums and cut into halves. Remove the pits and cut into small pieces. Set aside.

Now, combine strawberries, watermelon, banana, and plums in a juicer and process until juiced. Transfer to a serving glass and add some ice.

Serve immediately.

Nutritional information per serving: Kcal: 273, Protein: 5.1g, Carbs: 78.8g, Fats: 1.6g

18.   Zucchini Celery Juice

Ingredients:

1 small zucchini, sliced

1 cup of celery, chopped

1 cup of avocado, cubed

3 large radishes, chopped

1 cup of cucumber, sliced

¼ tsp of salt

1 oz of water

Preparation:

Wash the zucchini and cut into thin slices. Set aside.

Wash the celery and chop it into bite-sized pieces. Set aside.

Wash the cucumber and cut into thin slices. Fill the measuring cup and reserve the rest for later. Set aside.

Now, combine zucchini, celery, avocado, radishes, and cucumber in a juicer and process until juiced. Transfer to a serving glass and stir in the salt and water.

Serve cold.

Nutrition information per serving: Kcal: 235, Protein: 5.6g, Carbs: 22.3g, Fats: 22.6g

19. Brussels Sprout Zucchini Juice

Ingredients:

2 cups of Brussels sprouts, halved

1 small zucchini, chopped

1 cup of cucumber, sliced

2 large carrots, sliced

¼ tsp of turmeric, ground

Preparation:

Wash the Brussels sprouts and trim off the outer layers. Cut into halves and fill the measuring cups. Reserve the rest in the refrigerator.

Wash the zucchini and cut into thin slices. Set aside.

Wash the cucumber and cut into thin slices. Fill the measuring cup and reserve the rest for later.

Wash and peel the carrots. Cut into thin slices and set aside.

Now, combine Brussels sprouts, zucchini, radishes, cucumber, and carrots in a juicer and process until juiced.

Transfer to a serving glass and stir in the turmeric. Refrigerate for 15 minutes before serving.

Nutritional information per serving: Kcal: 118, Protein: 9.2g, Carbs: 35.7g, Fats: 1.3g

20.   Melon Raspberry Juice

Ingredients:

1 medium-sized wedge of honeydew melon

1 cup of raspberries

1 cup of spinach, chopped

1 small Golden Delicious apple, cored

¼ tsp of ginger, ground

Preparation:

Cut melon lengthwise in half. Scoop out the seeds and then wash the melon. Cut one wedge and peel it. Cut into bite-sized pieces and set aside. Reserve the rest in the refrigerator.

Place the raspberries in a colander and rinse well under cold running water. Drain and set aside.

Wash the spinach thoroughly under cold running water. Drain and chop into small pieces. Set aside.

Wash the apple and cut lengthwise in half. Remove the core and cut into bite-sized pieces. Set aside.

Now, combine melon, raspberries, spinach, and apple in a juicer and process until juiced. Transfer to a serving glass and stir in the ginger. Add some ice before serving.

Enjoy!

Nutritional information per serving: Kcal: 142, Protein: 4.5g, Carbs: 46.1g, Fats: 1.4g

21. Peach Apple Juice

Ingredients:

1 large peach, pitted and chopped

1 medium-sized green apple, cored and chopped

1 cup of watermelon, cubed

1 small banana, chunked

¼ tsp of cinnamon, ground

Preparation:

Wash the peach and cut lengthwise in half. Remove the pit and chop into bite-sized pieces. Set aside.

Wash the apple and cut in half. Remove the core and cut into bite-sized pieces. Set aside.

Cut the watermelon in half. Cut one large wedge and wrap the rest in a plastic foil and refrigerate. Peel the slice and cut into small cubes. Remove the pits and fill the measuring cup. Set aside.

Peel the banana and cut into small chunks. Set aside.

Now, combine peach, apple, watermelon, and banana in a juicer and process until juiced. Transfer to a serving glass and stir in the cinnamon.

Add some ice and serve immediately!

Nutrition information per serving: Kcal: 260, Protein: 4.4g, Carbs: 73.9g, Fats: 1.3g

22.   Sweet Avocado Mint Juice

Ingredients:

1 cup of avocado, pitted

1 cup of fresh mint, chopped

1 cup of strawberries, chopped

1 large apple, cored

1 large lemon, peeled

1 large cucumber, sliced

1 tbsp of liquid honey

1 oz of water

Preparation:

Peel the avocado and cut lengthwise in half. Remove the pit and cut into chunks and fill the measuring cup. Reserve the rest for later.

Wash the mint thoroughly and torn with hands. Set aside.

Wash the strawberries and cut into small pieces. Set aside.

Wash the apple and cut in half. Remove the core and cut into bite-sized pieces. Set aside.

Peel the lemon and cut lengthwise in half. Set aside.

Wash the cucumber and cut into thin slices. Set aside.

Now, combine avocado, mint, strawberries, lemon, and cucumber in a juicer and process until juiced. Transfer to serving glasses and stir in the water and honey. Add some ice and serve immediately.

Nutritional information per serving: Kcal: 376, Protein: 8.1g, Carbs: 67.8g, Fats: 23.3g

23.   Beet Spinach Juice

Ingredients:

1 cup of beets, sliced

1 cup of fresh spinach, torn

1 large red bell pepper, chopped

1 cup of purple cabbage, chopped

3 cherry tomatoes, halved

¼ tsp of salt

Preparation:

Wash the beets and trim off the green parts. Peel and cut into thin slices and fill the measuring cup. Reserve the rest for later.

Wash the bell pepper and cut lengthwise in half. Remove the stem and seeds. Cut into small pieces and set aside.

Combine cabbage and spinach in a large colander. Rinse thoroughly under cold running water and drain. Torn into small pieces and set aside.

Wash the cherry tomatoes and remove the stems. Cut into halves and set aside.

Now, combine bell pepper, cabbage, beets, spinach, and tomatoes in a juicer and process until juiced. Transfer to a serving glass and stir in the salt.

Serve immediately.

Nutrition information per serving: Kcal: 134, Protein: 11.5g, Carbs: 39.1g, Fats: 1.8g

24. Fennel Apple Juice

Ingredients:

1 cup of fennel, chopped

1 medium-sized Granny Smith's apple, cored

2 cups of broccoli, chopped

1 cup of fresh basil, chopped

1 oz of water

Preparation:

Trim off the fennel stalks and outer wilted layers. Wash and chop the fennel into bite-sized pieces. Fill the measuring cup and reserve the rest for later. Set aside.

Wash the apple and cut lengthwise in half. Remove the core and chop into small pieces. Set aside.

Wash the broccoli and trim off the outer leaves. Chop into small pieces and fill the measuring cup. Reserve the rest for later. Set aside.

Rinse the basil thoroughly under cold running water. Drain and torn into small pieces. Set aside.

Now, combine broccoli, fennel, apple, and basil in a juicer and process until juiced. Transfer to a serving glass and stir in the water.

Refrigerate for 10 minutes before serving.

Nutrition information per serving: Kcal: 140, Protein: 7.7g, Carbs: 41.8g, Fats: 1.3g

25. Zucchini Turmeric Juice

Ingredients:

1 medium-sized zucchini, sliced

1 cup of purple cabbage, torn

1 cup of celery, chopped

1 cup of cucumber, sliced

¼ tsp of ginger, ground

¼ tsp of turmeric, ground

¼ tsp of salt

Preparation:

Wash the zucchini and cut into thin slices. Set aside.

Rinse the purple cabbage under cold running water. Drain and torn into small pieces and set aside.

Wash the celery and chop into bite-sized pieces. Set aside.

Wash the cucumber and cut into slices. Fill the measuring cup and reserve the rest for later.

Now, combine cabbage, zucchini, celery, and cucumber in a juicer and process until juiced. Transfer to a serving glass and stir in the ginger, turmeric, and salt.

Refrigerate for 10 minutes before serving.

Nutrition information per serving: Kcal: 62, Protein: 4.7g, Carbs: 17.5g, Fats: 1g

26.   Cranberry Blackberry Juice

Ingredients:

1 cup of cranberries

1 cup of blackberries

1 cup of cantaloupe, diced

1 small Golden Delicious apple, cored

¼ tsp of cinnamon, ground

¼ tsp of ginger, ground

Preparation:

Combine cranberries and blackberries in a large colander. Rinse well under cold running water and drain. Set aside.

Cut the cantaloupe in half. Scrape out the seeds and cut one large wedge. Peel and dice into small pieces. Fill the measuring cup and wrap the rest in a plastic foil. Refrigerate for later.

Wash the apple cut lengthwise in half. Remove the core and cut into bite-sized pieces. Set aside.

Now, combine cranberries, blackberries, cantaloupe, and apple in a juicer and process until well juiced. Transfer to a serving glass and stir in the cinnamon and ginger.

Add some crushed ice and serve immediately.

Enjoy!

Nutrition information per serving: Kcal: 169, Protein: 4.1g, Carbs: 56.3g, Fats: 1.3g

27.   Squash Plum Juice

Ingredients:

1 cup of butternut squash, cubed

2 whole plums, pitted and chopped

1 cup of strawberries, chopped

1 medium-sized apple, cored

¼ tsp of ginger, ground

¼ tsp of turmeric, ground

Preparation:

Peel the butternut squash and cut lengthwise in half. Scoop out the seeds and wash the both halves. Cut into small cubes and fill the measuring cup. Wrap the rest of the squash in a plastic foil and refrigerate for later.

Wash the plums and cut in half. Remove the pits and cut into bite-sized pieces. Set aside.

Wash the strawberries and remove the stems. Cut into bite-sized pieces and fill the measuring cup. Reserve the rest in the refrigerator. Set aside.

Wash the apple and cut lengthwise in half. Remove the core and cut into bite-sized pieces. Set aside.

Now, combine strawberries, butternut squash, plum, and apple in a juicer and process until well juiced. Transfer to a serving glass and add some crushed ice.

Serve immediately.

Nutrition information per serving: Kcal: 214, Protein: 4.1g, Carbs: 65.2g, Fats: 1.2g

28.   Orange Spinach Juice

Ingredients:

1 large orange, peeled

½ cup of spinach, torn

1 cup of pineapple, chunked

3 Brussels sprouts, halved

1 oz of water

1 tsp of liquid honey

Preparation:

Peel the orange and divide into wedges. Cut each wedge in half and set aside.

Wash the spinach thoroughly under cold running water and torn with hands. Set aside.

Using a sharp paring knife, cut the top of the pineapple. Gently remove all hard skin and slice it into thin slices. Fill the measuring cup and reserve the rest for later.

Wash the Brussels sprouts and trim off the wilted leaves. Cut each in half and set aside.

Now, combine pineapple, orange, spinach, and Brussels sprouts in a juicer and process until well juiced. Transfer to a serving glass and stir in the honey and water.

Refrigerate for 10 minutes before serving.

Enjoy!

Nutrition information per serving: Kcal: 172, Protein: 7.9g, Carbs: 52.7g, Fats: 1.1g

29.   Carrot Collard Green Juice

Ingredients:

1 large carrot, chopped

1 cup of collard greens, torn

1 cup of avocado, chunked

1 cup of Romaine lettuce, shredded

1 whole cucumber, sliced

¼ tsp of ginger, ground

Preparation:

Wash and peel the carrot. Cut into thin slices and set aside.

Combine collard greens and lettuce in a large colander. Wash thoroughly under cold running water. Drain and shred. Set aside.

Peel the avocado and cut lengthwise in half. Remove the pit and cut into small chunks. Fill the measuring cup and reserve the rest in the refrigerator.

Wash the cucumber and cut into thin slices. Fill the measuring cup and reserve the rest for later. Set aside.

Now, combine carrot, collard greens, avocado, lettuce, and cucumber in a juicer and process until juiced. Transfer to a serving glass and stir in the ginger.

Refrigerate for 5 minutes before serving.

Nutrition information per serving: Kcal: 271, Protein: 7.3g, Carbs: 34.1g, Fats: 22.8g

30.   Lemon Spinach Juice

Ingredients:

1 cup of sweet potato, cubed

1 whole lemon, peeled

1 cup of fresh spinach, torn

1 cup of pomegranate seeds

2 oz of water

Preparation:

Peel the lemon and cut lengthwise In half. Set aside.

Wash the spinach thoroughly under cold running water. Drain and torn into small pieces. Set aside.

Peel the sweet potato and cut into small cubes. Place in a deep pot and add 3 cups of water. Bring it to a boil and cook for 5 minutes. Remove from the heat and drain. Set aside.

Cut the top of the pomegranate fruit using a sharp paring knife. Slice down to each of the white membranes inside of the fruit. Pop the seeds into a measuring cup and set aside.

Now, combine lemon, spinach, previously cooked potato, and pomegranate seeds in a juicer. Process until well juiced.

Transfer to a serving glass and stir in the water. Add some ice and serve immediately.

Enjoy!

Nutritional information per serving: Kcal: 195, Protein: 10.2g, Carbs: 56.1g, Fats: 2.1g

31.   Mustard Green Parsley Juice

Ingredients:

1 cup of mustard greens, torn

1 cup of parsley, torn

2 cups of Romaine lettuce, chopped

1 medium-sized Roma tomato, chopped

1 whole cucumber, sliced

¼ tsp of turmeric, ground

¼ tsp of salt

Preparation:

Combine mustard greens and parsley in a large colander. Rinse well and drain. Torn into small pieces and set aside.

Rinse the lettuce thoroughly under cold running water. Chop into small pieces and set aside.

Wash the tomato and place in a bowl. Chop into bite-sized pieces and reserve the tomato juice while cutting. Set aside.

Wash the cucumber and cut into thin slices. Set aside.

Now, combine lettuce, tomato, mustard greens, parsley, and cucumber in a juicer and process until juiced. Transfer to a serving glass and stir in the turmeric, salt, and reserved tomato juice.

Serve cold.

Nutrition information per serving: Kcal: 85, Protein: 7.6g, Carbs: 25.3g, Fats: 1.6g

32.   Lime Papaya Juice

Ingredients:

1 large lime, peeled

1 small papaya, seeded and peeled

1 cup of strawberries

1 cup of cranberries

3 oz of coconut water

Preparation:

Peel the lime and cut lengthwise in half. Set aside.

Peel the papaya and cut lengthwise in half. Scoop out the black seeds and flesh using a spoon. Cut into small chunks and set aside.

Place the strawberries and cranberries in a colander and wash under cold running water. Drain and set aside.

Now, process papaya, lime, strawberries, and cranberries in a juicer. Transfer to serving glasses and stir in the coconut water.

Add some ice, or refrigerate for 10 minutes before serving.

Enjoy!

Nutritional information per serving: Kcal: 153, Protein: 2.6g, Carbs: 50.9g, Fats: 1.8g

33.   Apple Strawberry Juice

Ingredients:

1 large red apple, cored

2 large strawberries, chopped

2 large grapefruits, peeled

1 small ginger knob, peeled

2 oz of coconut water

Preparation:

Wash the apple and cut in half. Remove the core and cut into bite-sized pieces. Set aside.

Wash the strawberries and cut into small pieces. Set aside.

Peel the grapefruits and divide into wedges. Set aside.

Peel the ginger knob and set aside.

Now, combine grapefruits, apple, strawberries, and ginger in a juicer. Process until well juiced and transfer to serving glasses. Stir in the coconut water and refrigerate for 10 minutes before serving.

Enjoy!

Nutritional information per serving: Kcal: 302, Protein: 4.8g, Carbs: 86.3g, Fats: 1.7g

34.   Apple Potato Juice

Ingredients:

1 medium-sized Golden Delicious apple, cored

1 cup of sweet potatoes, cubed

1 cup of celery, chopped

1 medium-sized orange, peeled

1 tbsp of fresh mint, torn

Preparation:

Wash the apple and cut lengthwise in half. Remove the core and cut into bite-sized pieces. Set aside.

Peel the sweet potato and cut into small cubes. Fill the measuring cup and reserve the rest for later. Set aside.

Wash the celery and cut into bite-sized pieces. Set aside.

Peel the orange and divide into wedges. Cut each wedge in half and set aside.

Now, combine sweet potatoes, celery, apple, and orange in a juicer. Process until well juiced. Transfer to a serving glass and sprinkle with mint.

Add some crushed ice and serve immediately.

Nutrition information per serving: Kcal: 236, Protein: 4.7g, Carbs: 67.8g, Fats: 0.7g

35.   Zucchini Lemon Juice

Ingredients:

1 medium-sized zucchini, chopped

1 whole lemon, peeled

1 cup of fresh kale, chopped

1 whole lime, peeled

1 cup of fresh mint, torn

Preparation:

Wash the zucchini and cut into small pieces. Set aside.

Peel the lemon and lime. Cut lengthwise in half and set aside.

Rinse the kale thoroughly under cold running water. Drain and chop into small pieces. Set aside.

Wash the mint and chop into small pieces. Set aside.

Now, combine zucchini, lemon, kale, lime, and mint in a juicer. Process until well juiced. Transfer to a serving glass and add some crushed ice.

Serve immediately.

Nutrition information per serving: Kcal: 79, Protein: 7g, Carbs: 24.7g, Fats: 1.7g

36.   Cucumber Artichoke Juice

Ingredients:

1 large cucumber

1 large artichoke head

1 cup of turnip greens

5 large asparagus spears

¼ tsp of ginger, ground

1 oz of water

Preparation:

Wash the cucumber and cut into thick slices. Set aside.

Using a sharp knife, trim off the outer leave of the artichoke. Cut into small pieces and set aside.

Wash the turnip greens and roughly chop it using hands. Set aside.

Wash the asparagus spears and trim off the woody ends. Cut into small pieces and set aside.

Now, process turnip greens, cucumber, artichoke, and asparagus in a juicer.

Transfer to serving glasses and stir in the ginger and water.

Add few ice cubes before serving.

Nutritional information per serving: Kcal: 101, Protein: 10.1g, Carbs: 35.8g, Fats: 0.8g

37.   Cantaloupe Cucumber Juice

Ingredients:

1 cup of cantaloupe, peeled and chopped

1 large cucumber

1 cup of avocado, peeled and pitted

1 large lemon, peeled

Preparation:

Cut the cantaloupe in half. Scoop out the seeds and flesh. Cut two wedges and peel them. Chop into chunks and set aside. Reserve the rest of the cantaloupe in a refrigerator.

Wash the cucumber and cut into thick slices. Set aside.

Peel the avocado and cut in half. Remove the pit and cut into chunks. Set aside.

Peel the lemon and cut in half. Set aside.

Now, process cantaloupe, cucumber, avocado, and lemon in a juicer.

Transfer to serving glasses and add some water to adjust the thickness, if needed.

Add some ice and serve immediately.

Nutritional information per serving: Kcal: 292, Protein: 6.8g, Carbs: 41.5g, Fats: 22.2g

38.   Ginger Carrot Juice

Ingredients:

1 large carrot, sliced

1 cup of pumpkin, cubed

1 cup of cucumber, sliced

1 large orange, peeled and wedged

1 small ginger knob, chopped

Preparation:

Wash and peel the carrot. Cut into thin slices and set aside.

Cut the top of a pumpkin. Cut lengthwise in half and then scrape out the seeds. Cut one large wedge and peel it. Cut into small cubes and fill the measuring cup. Reserve the rest in the refrigerator.

Wash the cucumber and cut into thin slices. Fill the measuring cup and reserve the rest for later. Set aside.

Peel the orange and divide into wedges. Cut each wedge in half and set aside.

Peel the ginger knob and cut into small pieces. Set aside.

Now, combine pumpkin, carrot, cucumber, orange, and ginger in a juicer. Process until well juiced. Transfer to a serving glass and add some ice.

Serve immediately.

Nutrition information per serving: Kcal: 130, Protein: 4.1g, Carbs: 39.1g, Fats: 0.6g

39. Lettuce Cabbage Juice

Ingredients:

1 cup of red leaf lettuce, chopped

1 cup of purple cabbage, chopped

1 medium-sized artichoke, chopped

1 cup of fresh basil, torn

1 cup of cucumber, sliced

1 large carrot, sliced

Preparation:

Combine lettuce and cabbage in a large colander and rinse well under cold running water. Drain and chop into small pieces. Set aside.

Trim off the outer layers of the artichoke using a sharp paring knife. Cut into bite-sized pieces and set aside.

Rinse the basil with cold water and torn into small pieces. Set aside.

Wash the cucumber and cut into thin slices. Fill the measuring cup and reserve the rest in the refrigerator.

Wash and peel the carrot. Cut into thin slices and set aside.

Now, combine artichoke, basil, lettuce, cabbage, cucumber, and carrot in a juicer and process until juiced.

Transfer to a serving glass and serve immediately.

Nutritional information per serving: Kcal: 88, Protein: 7.6g, Carbs: 30.1g, Fats: 0.7g

40.   Basil Cucumber Juice

Ingredients:

1 cup of fresh basil, torn

1 cup of cucumber, sliced

1 medium-sized zucchini, chopped

1 cup of red leaf lettuce, torn

1 cup of avocado, cut into bite-sized pieces

Preparation:

Combine basil and lettuce in a large colander and rinse under cold running water. Drain and torn with hands into small pieces. Set aside.

Wash the cucumber and cut into thin slices. Fill the measuring cup and refrigerate for later.

Peel the zucchini and chop into small pieces. Set aside.

Peel the avocado and cut lengthwise in half. Remove the pit and cut into bite-sized pieces. Fill the measuring cup and reserve the rest in the refrigerator.

Now, combine zucchini, basil, lettuce, avocado, and cucumber in a juicer. Process until well juiced. Transfer to a serving glass and add some ice.

Serve immediately.

Nutrition information per serving: Kcal: 234, Protein: 6.7g, Carbs: 21.7g, Fats: 22.3g

41.   Celery Leek Juice

Ingredients:

1 cup of celery, chopped

1 whole leek, chopped

2 cups of parsley, torn

1 whole cucumber, sliced

1 cup of beet greens, torn

¼ tsp of turmeric powder, ground

¼ tsp of cumin, ground

Preparation:

Wash the celery and chop into small pieces. Fill the measuring cup and reserve the rest in the refrigerator. Set aside.

Wash the leek and chop into bite-sized pieces. Set aside.

Combine parsley and beet greens in a large colander. Rinse well under cold running water and drain. Torn into small pieces and set aside.

Wash the cucumber and cut into thin slices. Set aside.

Now, combine celery, leek, parsley, beet greens, and cucumber in a juicer and process until juiced. Transfer to a serving glass and stir in the turmeric and cumin.

Serve immediately.

Nutrition information per serving: Kcal: 127, Protein: 8.4g, Carbs: 35.7g, Fats: 1.7g

42. Cucumber Banana Juice

Ingredients:

1 cup of cucumber, sliced

1 medium-sized banana, sliced

1 small Granny Smith's apple, cored

1 tbsp of aloe juice

1 large celery stalk, chopped

Preparation:

Wash the cucumber and cut into thin slices. Fill the measuring cup and reserve the rest for later. Set aside.

Peel the banana and cut into chunks. Set aside.

Wash the apple and cut in half. Remove the core and cut into bite-sized pieces. Set aside.

Wash the celery stalk and chop into bite-sized pieces. Set aside.

Now, combine cucumber, banana, apple, and celery in a juicer. Process until juiced.

Transfer to a serving glass and stir in the aloe juice.

Add some crushed ice and serve immediately.

Nutrition information per serving: Kcal: 174, Protein: 2.7g, Carbs: 50.3g, Fats: 0.8g

43.   Onion Pepper Juice

Ingredients:

1 medium-sized spring onion

1 large bell pepper, seeded

1 cup of cherry tomatoes

1 garlic clove, peeled

¼ tsp of Cayenne pepper, ground

¼ tsp of salt

A handful of fresh cilantro

Preparation:

Wash the spring onion and chop into small pieces. Set aside.

Wash the bell pepper and cut in half. Remove the seeds and chop into small pieces. Set aside.

Wash the cherry tomatoes and place them in a bowl. Cut in half and reserve the juice while cutting. Set aside.

Peel the garlic and set aside.

Wash the cilantro thoroughly and torn with hands.

Set aside.

Now, combine tomatoes, spring onion, cilantro, bell pepper, and garlic in a juicer and process until juiced.

Transfer to serving glasses and stir in Cayenne pepper and salt.

Refrigerate for 5 minutes and serve.

Nutritional information per serving: Kcal: 41, Protein: 2.8g, Carbs: 11.5g, Fats: 0.6g

44.   Celery Grapefruit Juice

Ingredients:

1 cup of celery, chopped

1 whole grapefruit, peeled

2 large carrots, chunked

1 small Golden Delicious apple, cored and chopped

¼ tsp of cinnamon, ground

Preparation:

Wash the celery and cut into small pieces. Fill the measuring cup and reserve the rest in the refrigerator.

Peel the grapefruit and divide into wedges. Cut each wedge in half and set aside.

Wash and peel the carrots. Cut into small chunks and set aside.

Wash the apple and cut lengthwise in half. Remove the core and cut into bite-sized pieces. Set aside.

Now, combine celery, grapefruit, carrots, and apple in a juicer and process until well juiced. Transfer to a serving glass and stir in the cinnamon.

Add some crushed ice and serve immediately.

Enjoy!

Nutritional information per serving: Kcal: 203, Protein: 4.3g, Carbs: 60.6g, Fats: 1.1g

ADDITIONAL TITLES FROM THIS AUTHOR

70 Effective Meal Recipes to Prevent and Solve Being Overweight: Burn Fat Fast by Using Proper Dieting and Smart Nutrition

By

Joe Correa CSN

48 Acne Solving Meal Recipes: The Fast and Natural Path to Fixing Your Acne Problems in Less Than 10 Days!

By

Joe Correa CSN

41 Alzheimer's Preventing Meal Recipes: Reduce or Eliminate Your Alzheimer's Condition in 30 Days or Less!

By

Joe Correa CSN

70 Effective Breast Cancer Meal Recipes: Prevent and Fight Breast Cancer with Smart Nutrition and Powerful Foods

By

Joe Correa CSN

www.ingramcontent.com/pod-product-compliance
Lightning Source LLC
Chambersburg PA
CBHW030249030426
42336CB00009B/304